SMOOTHIES FOR ULCER MANAGEMENT:

Smooth Your Way to Ulcer With These Nutritious Smoothie Recipes

JANET MARTINS

Contents

DISCLAIMER:

All content is provided as general information only, and should not be taken as medical advice or professional guidance. Please consult with a qualified healthcare provider if you have any questions or concerns about your individual situation.

INTRODUCTION

Are you looking for a nutritious way to manage your ulcers? If so, consider trying out some smoothies! Smoothies are a great way to get all the nutrients your body needs, and they can be especially helpful if you are struggling with ulcer management. In this book, we will discuss the benefits of smoothies for ulcer management and provide some recipes for you to try out!

Living with an ulcer can be difficult, but it doesn't have to be. With these nutritious smoothie recipes, you can help soothe your ulcer and improve your overall health! These recipes are packed with vitamins, minerals, and antioxidants that will help speed up the healing process. So what are you waiting for? Start blending!

If you're looking for a nutritious way to manage your ulcers, look no further than these delicious smoothie recipes! These recipes are packed with antioxidants, vitamins, and minerals that will help speed up the healing process. Plus, they're all incredibly tasty and easy to make. So why not give them a try?

PART 1

INTRODUCTION TO ULCER MANAGEMENT

WHAT IS AN ULCER?

Ulcers are wounds that either take a long time to heal or continually come back. They may manifest themselves in various ways, and they can do so both on your body's exterior and inside.

They may be located in areas of your body that are visible to you, such as an ulcer on the skin of your thigh, or they can be found in areas that are not visible to you, such as an ulcer in the lining of your stomach or upper intestine that is peptic.

You may acquire them anywhere, from your eye to your foot.

Accidents, illnesses, and infections are all potential triggers for them. Their appearance varies according to where you have them and how you obtained them. While some may clear up independently, others can lead to significant complications if they are not treated.

Ulcers are open wounds on the stomach lining or the small intestine. You may also have sores on your esophagus (throat). The small intestine is home to the majority of people's ulcers. These sores are referred to as ulcers of the duodenum. Gastric ulcers are another name for stomach ulcers. Esophageal ulcers are another name for ulcers that are located in the throat.

causes of ulcer

1. pylori bacteria

It's common to have an H. pylori infection, and it's usually harmless for most people.

But sometimes, it causes ulcers in the stomach (gastric ulcer) or duodenum (duodenal ulcer).

It's not clear exactly why some people are more affected than others.

Anti-inflammatory medicines (NSAIDs)

NSAIDs are medicines widely used to treat pain, high temperature (fever), and inflammation (swelling).

Commonly used NSAIDs include:

- ibuprofen
- aspirin
- naproxen
- diclofenac

Many people take NSAIDs without having any side effects. But there's always a risk the medication could cause problems, such as stomach ulcers, particularly if taken for a long time or at high doses.

You may be advised not to take NSAIDs if you currently have or have had a stomach ulcer.

Lifestyle factors

There is not much evidence to suggest that certain aspects of one's lifestyle, such as eating spicy foods, experiencing stress, or drinking alcohol, might induce stomach ulcers. Yet, they can make your symptoms much more severe.

It is believed that smoking might reduce the effectiveness of therapy for stomach ulcers and increase the chance of getting ulcers in the stomach.

Helicobacter pylori are responsible for the majority of ulcers (H. pylori). This is an infection caused by bacteria. The acidity of the meals we consume has the potential to aggravate both the pain and the discomfort. Ulcers are also often brought on by using anti-inflammatory drugs like ibuprofen or aspirin for an extended period of time. Both stress and meals that are very spicy might make an ulcer worse.

SYMPTOMS OF ULCERS

Common ulcer symptoms include:

- Discomfort between meals or during the night (duodenal ulcer)
- Discomfort when you eat or drink (gastric ulcer)
- Stomach pain that wakes you up at night
- Feel full fast
- Bloating, burning, or dull pain in your stomach
- Comes and goes days or weeks at a time

- The discomfort lasts for minutes or hours

If your ulcer becomes perforated (torn), it becomes bleeding. This can cause the following symptoms:

- Nausea
- Vomiting blood
- Unexpected weight loss
- Blood in your stool or dark stools
- Pain in your back

TREATMENT FOR ULCER

You are not recommended to treat an ulcer on your own before consulting with a medical professional. Antacids and acid blockers available over the counter may alleviate some or all of the discomfort, but the respite they provide is always temporary. On the other hand, you may discover relief from ulcer discomfort and a treatment that will last a lifetime with the assistance of a medical professional.

The therapy for ulcers focuses mostly on lowering the amount of acid produced by the stomach and strengthening the protective lining in direct contact with stomach acids. These are the two primary aims of ulcer treatment. Your doctor will also treat the bacterial infection if it is determined that it is the cause of your ulcer.

MEDICATIONS

Medications are usually used to treat mild-to-moderate ulcers.

- **Antibiotics**. If H. pylori bacteria cause your ulcer, antibiotics can cure the ulcer. Usually, the doctor will prescribe triple or quadruple therapy, which combines several antibiotics with heartburn drugs.

- **Triple therapy combines** two antibiotics, amoxicillin, and clarithromycin, with a proton pump inhibitor. The doctor can substitute metronidazole (Flagyl) for amoxicillin if you're allergic to penicillin. If you've had repeated bouts of these antibiotics or live in an area with resistance to clarithromycin or metronidazole, quadruple therapy treatment with two antibiotics (like metronidazole and tetracycline) plus bismuth and a proton-pump inhibitor works best. No matter the plan, you should take all medications for 10-14 days.

- **Proton pump inhibitors.** PPIs are acid reducers. These medications include esomeprazole (Nexium) and omeprazole (Prilosec).

- **H2 blockers.** These medicines are also called histamine receptor blockers or H2-receptor antagonists. They block a natural chemical called histamine, which tells your stomach to make acid. H2 blockers include cimetidine (Tagamet), famotidine (Pepcid), and nizatidine (Axid).

- **Bismuth**. This medication covers the ulcer and protects it from stomach acid. It can also help kill *H. pylori* infections. Doctors usually prescribe it with antibiotics.

- **Antacids**. They may ease your symptoms for a short time, but they don't treat ulcers. Taking an antacid can also keep antibiotics from working. Talk to your doctor before taking an antacid for peptic ulcer disease.

SURGERY

Your doctor may recommend surgery if you have a severe ulcer that keeps returning despite taking medicine to treat it and if the ulcer does not improve.

If you have a bleeding ulcer, you must undergo an emergency operation (also called a hemorrhaging ulcer). First, the surgeon will locate the cause of the bleeding, often a tiny artery near the base of the ulcer, and then they will repair it. For example, suppose you have a perforated ulcer or perforations in the wall of your stomach or duodenum. In that case, you will need urgent surgery to repair the damage (the first part of your small intestine).

Some individuals choose surgery to reduce the quantity of stomach acid their body produces. Have a detailed conversation with your physician about the potential risks involved before you go forward with that plan. It is possible that your ulcer could return, that it will create issues with your liver, or that you will develop dumping syndrome, which is characterized by persistent stomach discomfort, diarrhea, vomiting, or sweating after consuming food.

ALTERNATIVE TREATMENTS

Although alternative therapies have been shown to relieve symptoms, you should only use them as supplements to conventional treatment.

PART 2

THE BENEFITS OF SMOOTHIES FOR ULCER PREVENTION AND TREATMENT

NUTRITIONAL BENEFITS OF SMOOTHIES

1 – Hydration all day long

Smoothies contain a high percentage of water, so they will help you stay hydrated longer. Try it for breakfast… you'll notice its benefits all day long!

2 – No more snacking between meals!

Smoothies are the perfect meal replacement: They not only will keep you satiated and away from unhealthy snacks, but they also have the potential to help you slim down! With a wide range of fruits and veggies in each glass, these drinks make it easier than ever to cut calories while staying fuller for longer. So say goodbye to mid-day cravings and hello to smoothie power - your body will thank you for it!

3 – Lighter digestion

Combining all the ingredients in a blender produces digestible enzymes that aid your body to absorb essential vitamins and micronutrients. Combined with its high fiber content, this allows for rapid nutrient absorption and an easier digestion experience.

4 – They accelerate your metabolism and detoxify your body

Not only is fiber incredibly helpful, but it can also accelerate your metabolism! If you've recently become active and desire to achieve quick results, smoothies will certainly aid in burning fat while simultaneously boosting muscle building. In addition, these delicious fruit & veggie combos also contain minerals that flush out the system - making you feel younger and fitter than ever!

5 – Full of energy!

Enjoying a smoothie has an abundance of benefits, particularly because it is a liquid-based food. This means your body immediately absorbs the minerals, antioxidants, and vitamins - giving you that necessary burst of energy to last throughout your day!

6 – They improve your mental health and your performance

The hustle and bustle of life often lead to us consuming fast, heavy meals that lack the vital nutrients our body needs - leading us into a state of sluggishness, both physically and mentally. As a result, it becomes harder for you to focus and stay energized throughout the day.

With a variety of vitamins and minerals, smoothies made from healthful fruits and vegetables offer protection against various ailments while also aiding overall well-being. For example, consider coconut-based beverages; they're high in fiber, and magnesium, yet low in sugar - perfect for enhancing memory and activating the brain more efficiently!

7 – Your skin will be glowing!

The nourishing natural ingredients cleanse your body of toxins and other impurities and are also an excellent source of antioxidants. In addition, these nutrients will help to promote the regeneration process of your skin's cells for a youthful, blemish-free appearance that endures.

8 – Recover better after exercise

Smoothies are the perfect companion for any athlete. After a workout, they replenish all the hydration, salts, and minerals your body needs to recover from physical activity properly. Additionally, you can consume them as a nutritious snack before exercising; this will provide your body with an abundance of energy so that you can reach every goal!

9 – Drinking a smoothie a day... keeps the doctor away

The vitamins and antioxidants in smoothies are very important for your immune system. They are also a great source of minerals, which will help make your bones stronger and healthier.

HOW TO MAKE AN EFFECTIVE SMOOTHIE FOR ULCER PREVENTION AND TREATMENT

1 . Choose a high-fiber base: Start with a fiber-rich base like oats, barley, wheat germ, or flaxseed. These are all great sources of dietary fiber which helps to bulk up the smoothie and can help reduce symptoms of ulcers by soothing the inflamed tissue in the digestive tract.

2. Add fruits and vegetables: Next, add some fresh or frozen fruits and vegetables to the mix. Fruits such as strawberries, kiwi fruit, apples, oranges, grapes, and blueberries are all good sources of antioxidants and vitamins supporting ulcer prevention and treatment. Dark leafy greens such as spinach, kale, and chard are also excellent additions because they contain anti-inflammatory compounds that can soothe the digestive tract.

3. Include some healthy fats: Healthy fats are essential for overall health and can also help reduce symptoms of ulcers. Avocados, nuts and seeds, coconut oil, and olive oil are good options for your smoothie.

4. Add protein: Protein is important for repairing cells damaged by ulcers and other digestive issues. Good protein sources to add to a smoothie include Greek yogurt, cottage cheese, almond butter, or hemp seeds.

5 . Blend it up: Once you have all your ingredients ready, blend them into a blender or food processor until everything is combined into a delicious smoothie. Then, sip it immediately for the best results!

6 . Enjoy: Drink your smoothie daily to help reduce symptoms of existing ulcers and protect against future issues. Ulcers can be painful, but

you can keep them under control with the right nutrition and a healthy lifestyle!

COMMON INGREDIENTS USED IN MAKING SMOOTHIES FOR ULCER PREVENTION AND TREATMENT

1 . Fruits contain important vitamins and minerals essential for proper healing and ulcer prevention. Bananas, blueberries, raspberries, strawberries, peaches, mangos, apples, and other fruits can be added to smoothies to provide much-needed nutrition.

2. Leafy Greens – Leafy greens like kale, spinach, collard greens, and romaine lettuce are filled with essential nutrients that help support the body's natural digestive system health. Adding these leafy greens to a smoothie can help reduce

inflammation associated with existing ulcers while protecting future issues.

3. Yogurt – Yogurt is an excellent source of probiotics that help restore beneficial bacteria in the gut, thus promoting overall digestive health. Plain yogurt is best for a smoothie as it provides healthy bacteria without extra sugars or preservatives.

4. Almond Butter – Almond butter is a great source of healthy fats which can help reduce inflammation and improve digestion. Adding almond butter to your smoothie will provide essential vitamins, minerals, and fiber for overall digestive health and ulcer prevention.

5. Hemp Seeds – Hemp seeds are an excellent source of omega-3 fatty acids, beneficial in treating and preventing ulcers. They also provide protein, fiber, magnesium, calcium, iron, and other essential nutrients that support the body's natural healing process. Adding hemp seeds to

your smoothie is an easy way to get all their benefits.

6 . Ginger – Ginger has been used for centuries to help alleviate digestive issues and reduce inflammation in the body. Adding ginger to your smoothie can help soothe existing ulcers while protecting future issues.

7 . Turmeric is a powerful anti-inflammatory that helps soothe the digestive system and reduce symptoms of existing ulcers. Adding turmeric to your smoothie can also provide antioxidants and other essential nutrients for overall digestive health.

8 . Apple Cider Vinegar – Apple cider vinegar is a powerful tool for restoring digestive health and supporting the body's natural healing process. Adding a tablespoon of apple cider vinegar to your smoothie can help reduce inflammation, improve digestion, and provide essential vitamins and minerals necessary for ulcer prevention.

9 . Flax Seeds – Flax seeds are an excellent source of dietary fiber which helps maintain a healthy digestive system. They also contain omega-3 fatty acids and other essential vitamins and minerals that can help reduce inflammation and provide protection against future ulcers. Adding flax seeds to your smoothie is an easy way to get all their benefits.

10 . Coconut Water – Coconut water is a great source of electrolytes and other essential nutrients for maintaining digestive health. Adding coconut water to your smoothie can help soothe existing ulcers while protecting future issues.

TIPS FOR MANAGING ULCERS

Mind Your Meds

The majority of patients who suffer from stomach ulcers use medications that are prescribed to them to lessen the discomfort and speed up the healing process. Antibiotics, for instance, are effective against H. pylori bacterial infections, the most common cause of stomach ulcers. On the other hand, antibiotics and other medications will not be as effective if you do not take them exactly as directed. It is best to take acid blockers on an empty stomach first thing in the morning, then again 30 minutes before meals. If your physician provides medication for your stomach ulcer, take it precisely as directed on the label. And make sure you complete the prescribed amount of the medication, even if you start to feel better.

Avoid Antacids

Antacids, such as Tums, can help your stomach ulcer feel better for a little while. But you should avoid taking them. Antacids won't heal a stomach ulcer and can interfere with medications that do. For example, antacids reduce how well some antibiotics work.

Don't Overdo Dairy

Some people believe that drinking milk can help cure a stomach ulcer. And while it's true that milk can make you feel better briefly, it isn't a cure for ulcers. Drinking too much milk can increase stomach acid, worsening an ulcer.

Kick the Habit

Smoking slows the healing process. It can also make an ulcer worse. In addition, smoking after you heal from an ulcer can cause the ulcer to return. Smoking's effect on ulcers is just one more reason to quit. Ask your doctor for resources that can help you kick the habit.

Reconsider Your Pain Pills

Nonsteroidal anti-inflammatory drugs (NSAIDs), a pain reliever, are the second-most common cause of stomach ulcers. NSAIDs include aspirin (Bayer), ibuprofen (Advil and Motrin), and naproxen (Aleve). If you take NSAIDs, ask your doctor if you can take another pain reliever instead. If NSAIDs are necessary, ask about "enteric coated" medications that can help protect the lining of your stomach. And try to take the pain pills with a meal.

Enjoy Your Diet

Many people think that spicy foods can cause an ulcer. Not so. Although spicy foods can irritate ulcer symptoms in some people, there's no special diet you must follow if you have stomach ulcers. So enjoy your food—but watch your drink. Drinking alcohol slows the healing of ulcers and can make them worse.

Know When to Get Help

Sometimes stomach ulcers lead to problems that require immediate treatment. These symptoms include quick or heavy bleeding. Signs that your ulcer may be bleeding include black, sticky stools or blood in the stool, vomit that looks like coffee

grounds or contains blood, or feeling light-
headed.

PART 3:

20 RECIPES FOR ULCER MANAGEMENT WITH DIRECTIONS

FRUIT SMOOTHIES

Strawberry Smoothie

ingredient

-1 cup frozen strawberries

-1/2 cup plain nonfat Greek yogurt

-1/4 cup orange juice

-1 tablespoon honey

-Ice cubes (optional)

Directions:

Combine all the ingredients in a blender. Blend until smooth. Serve immediately.

Banana Smoothie

ingredient

-1 frozen banana

-1/2 cup plain nonfat Greek yogurt

-1 tablespoon chia seeds

-1/4 cup almond milk (or other non-dairy milk)

-Ice cubes (optional)

Directions:

Combine all the ingredients in a blender. Blend until smooth. Serve immediately.

Mango Smoothie

ingredient

-1 cup frozen mango cubes

-1/2 cup plain nonfat Greek yogurt

-1 tablespoon flaxseeds

-1/4 cup orange juice

-Ice cubes (optional)

Directions:

Combine all the ingredients in a blender. Blend until smooth. Serve immediately.

Blueberry Smoothie

ingredient

-1 cup frozen blueberries

-1/2 cup plain nonfat Greek yogurt

-1 tablespoon almond butter

-1/4 cup apple juice

-Ice cubes (optional)

Directions:

Combine all the ingredients in a blender. Blend until smooth. Serve immediately.

Pear Smoothie

ingredient

-1 cup frozen pear cubes

-1/2 cup plain nonfat Greek yogurt

-1 tablespoon sunflower seeds

-1/4 cup coconut milk (or other dairy-free milk)

-Ice cubes (optional)

Directions:

Combine all the ingredients in a blender. Blend until smooth. Serve immediately.

Perfect Berry Smoothie

ingredient

-1/2 cup frozen strawberries

-1/2 cup frozen blueberries

-1/2 cup plain nonfat Greek yogurt

-1 tablespoon chia seeds

-1/4 cup almond milk (or other dairy-free milk)

-Ice cubes (optional)

Directions:

Combine all the ingredients in a blender. Blend until smooth. Serve immediately. Enjoy!

This delicious and nutritious berry smoothie is perfect for ulcer prevention and management as it contains vitamin C, antioxidants, and probiotics. Vitamin C helps boost the immune system, while antioxidants help fight free radical damage that can lead to ulcer symptoms.

Green Smoothie

ingredient

-1 cup spinach

-1/2 cucumber

-1/2 cup plain nonfat Greek yogurt

-1 tablespoon flaxseeds

-1/4 cup orange juice

-Ice cubes (optional)

Directions:

Combine all the ingredients in a blender. Blend until smooth. Serve immediately. Enjoy!

Pineapple Smoothie

ingredient

-1 cup frozen pineapple cubes

-1/2 banana

-1/2 cup plain nonfat Greek yogurt

-1 tablespoon almond butter

-1/4 cup coconut milk (or other dairy-free milk)

-Ice cubes (optional)

Directions:

Combine all the ingredients in a blender. Blend until smooth. Serve immediately. Enjoy!

Peach Smoothie

ingredient

-1 cup frozen peaches

-1/2 banana

-1/2 cup plain nonfat Greek yogurt

-1 tablespoon chia seeds

-1/4 cup almond milk (or other dairy-free milk)

-Ice cubes (optional)

Directions:

Combine all the ingredients in a blender. Blend until smooth. Serve immediately. Enjoy!

Orange Smoothie

ingredient

-1 cup frozen orange slices

-1/2 banana

-1/2 cup plain nonfat Greek yogurt

-1 tablespoon flaxseeds

-1/4 cup coconut milk (or other dairy-free milk)

-Ice cubes (optional)

Directions:

Combine all the ingredients in a blender. Blend until smooth. Serve immediately.

Raspberry Smoothie

ingredient

-1 cup frozen raspberries

-1/2 banana

-1/2 cup plain nonfat Greek yogurt

-1 tablespoon chia seeds

-1/4 cup almond milk (or other dairy-free milk)

-Ice cubes (optional)

Directions:

Combine all the ingredients in a blender. Blend until smooth. Serve immediately.

Grape Smoothie

ingredient

-1 cup frozen grapes

-1/2 banana

-1/2 cup plain nonfat Greek yogurt

-1 tablespoon ground flaxseed

-1/4 cup coconut milk (or other dairy-free milk)

-Ice cubes (optional)

Directions:

Combine all the ingredients in a blender. Blend until smooth. Serve immediately.

Chocolate Strawberry Smoothie

ingredient

-1 cup frozen strawberries

-1/2 banana

-1/2 cup plain nonfat Greek yogurt

-1 tablespoon cocoa powder

-1/4 cup almond milk (or other dairy-free milk)

-Ice cubes (optional)

Directions:

Combine all the ingredients in a blender. Blend until smooth. Serve immediately. Enjoy!

Green Apple Smoothie

ingredient

-1 cup frozen green apple slices

-1/2 banana

-1/2 cup plain nonfat Greek yogurt

-1 tablespoon chia seeds

-1/4 cup coconut milk (or other dairy-free milk)

-Ice cubes (optional)

Directions:

Combine all the ingredients in a blender. Blend until smooth. Serve immediately. Which can help manage existing ulcers.

Blueberry Pineapple Smoothie

ingredient

-1 cup frozen blueberries

-1/2 cup pineapple chunks

-1/2 banana

-1/2 cup plain nonfat Greek yogurt

-1 tablespoon ground flaxseed

-1/4 cup almond milk (or other dairy-free milk)

-Ice cubes (optional)

Directions:

Combine all the ingredients in a blender. Blend until smooth. Serve immediately.

Mango Avocado Smoothie

ingredient

-1 cup frozen mango chunks

-1/2 ripe avocado

-1/2 banana

-1/2 cup plain nonfat Greek yogurt

-1 tablespoon hemp seeds

-1/4 cup coconut milk (or other dairy-free milk)

-Ice cubes (optional)

Directions:

Combine all the ingredients in a blender. Blend until smooth. Serve immediately.

Acai Berry Smoothie

ingredient

-1 cup frozen acai berries

-1/2 banana

-1/2 cup plain nonfat Greek yogurt

-1 tablespoon flaxseeds

-1/4 cup almond milk (or other dairy-free milk)

-Ice cubes (optional)

Directions:

Combine all the ingredients in a blender. Blend until smooth. Serve immediately.

Cinnamon Apple Smoothie

ingredient

-1 cup frozen apple slices

-1/2 banana

-1/2 cup plain nonfat Greek yogurt

-1 tablespoon ground cinnamon

-1/4 cup coconut milk (or other dairy-free milk)

-Ice cubes (optional)

Directions:

Combine all the ingredients in a blender. Blend until smooth. Serve immediately. Enjoy!

Smoothies are an easy and delicious way to get important nutrients into your diet that can help reduce symptoms of existing ulcers and protect against future issues. Make sure to drink them regularly for the best results!

Watermelon Smoothie

ingredient

-1 cup frozen watermelon chunks

-1/2 banana

-1/2 cup plain nonfat Greek yogurt

-1 tablespoon chia seeds

-1/4 cup almond milk (or other dairy-free milk)

-Ice cubes (optional)

Directions:

Combine all the ingredients in a blender. Blend until smooth. Serve immediately. Enjoy!

Watermelon is rich in vitamins and minerals that can help support the body's natural healing process, making it an ideal ingredient for ulcer prevention and treatment. Adding this delicious fruit to your regular smoothie routine can help keep you feeling healthy and strong while helping to manage existing or prevent future ulcers.

Kiwi Smoothie

ingredient

-1 cup frozen kiwi slices

-1/2 banana

-1/2 cup plain nonfat Greek yogurt

-1 tablespoon hemp seeds

-1/4 cup coconut milk (or other dairy-free milk)

-Ice cubes (optional)

Directions:

Combine all the ingredients in a blender. Blend until smooth. Serve immediately. Enjoy!

Kiwis are rich in Vitamin C and have natural antihistamine properties that can help to reduce inflammation associated with ulcers, making it a great addition to your smoothie routine. Regularly drinking this nutritious fruit will provide you with essential vitamins and minerals that can help combat existing or prevent future issues.

Dragon Fruit Smoothie

ingredient

-1 cup frozen dragon fruit

-1/2 banana

-1/2 cup plain nonfat Greek yogurt

-1 tablespoon ground cinnamon

-1/4 cup almond milk (or other dairy-free milk)

-Ice cubes (optional)

Directions:

Combine all the ingredients in a blender. Blend until smooth. Serve immediately. Enjoy!

Dragon fruit is packed with antioxidants and other important vitamins and minerals that can help reduce inflammation and support healing, making it an ideal ingredient for ulcer prevention and treatment. Adding this delicious fruit to your regular smoothie routine can help keep you healthy and strong while helping to manage existing or prevent future ulcers.

Grapefruit Smoothie

ingredient

-1 cup frozen grapefruit slices

-1/2 banana

-1/2 cup plain nonfat Greek yogurt

-1 tablespoon chia seeds

-1/4 cup coconut milk (or other dairy-free milk)

-Ice cubes (optional)

Directions:

Combine all the ingredients in a blender. Blend until smooth. Serve immediately. Enjoy!

Grapefruits are packed with Vitamin C and have natural antihistamine properties that can help to reduce inflammation associated with ulcers, making it a great addition to your smoothie routine.

Cantaloupe Smoothie

ingredient

-1 cup frozen cantaloupe chunks

-1/2 banana

-1/2 cup plain nonfat Greek yogurt

-1 tablespoon hemp seeds

-1/4 cup almond milk (or other dairy-free milk)

-Ice cubes (optional)

Directions:

Combine all the ingredients in a blender. Blend until smooth. Serve immediately. Enjoy!

Cantaloupes are packed with vitamins and minerals that can help support the body's natural healing process, making them an ideal ingredient for ulcer prevention and treatment.

Honeydew Smoothie

ingredients

-1 cup frozen honeydew chunks

-1/2 banana

-1/2 cup plain nonfat Greek yogurt

-1 tablespoon ground cinnamon

-1/4 cup coconut milk (or other dairy-free milk)

-Ice cubes (optional)

Directions:

Combine all the ingredients in a blender. Blend until smooth. Serve immediately. Enjoy!

Honeydews are rich in Vitamin C and have natural antihistamine properties that can help to reduce inflammation associated with ulcers, making it a great addition to your smoothie routine.

VEGETABLE SMOOTHIES

Spinach Smoothie

Ingredient:

1 cup spinach

1 ripe banana

1/2 cup plain Greek yogurt

3/4 cup orange juice

1 teaspoon lemon juice

2 tablespoons honey (optional)

Instructions:

1. Wash and dry the spinach leaves.

2. Peel and chop the banana, then add to a blender with the spinach, yogurt, orange juice, and lemon juice. Blend until smooth.

3. Taste-test the smoothie and add honey if desired; blend again.

4. Pour into glasses and enjoy!

This delicious spinach smoothie is an easy way to get essential nutrients that can help protect against ulcers and soothe existing ones.

Carrot Smoothie

Ingredient:

2 large carrots

1/2 cup plain Greek yogurt

1 teaspoon honey (optional)

3/4 cup almond milk

1 tablespoon lemon juice

Instructions:

1. Wash and peel the carrots, then cut them into small pieces.

2. Add the carrots to a blender and the yogurt, honey (if desired), almond milk, and lemon juice. Blend until smooth.

3. Taste-test the smoothie and add more honey if desired; blend again.

4. Pour into glasses and enjoy!

Beet Smoothie

Ingredients:

1 small beet

1 ripe banana

1/2 cup plain Greek yogurt

3/4 cup almond milk

2 tablespoons honey (optional)

Instructions:

1. Wash and peel the beet, then cut it into small pieces.

2. Peel and chop the banana, then add to a blender with the beet, yogurt, almond milk, and honey (if desired). Blend until smooth.

3. Taste-test the smoothie and add more honey if desired; blend again.

4. Pour into glasses and enjoy!

This refreshing beet smoothie is packed with nutrients that can help reduce inflammation in your digestive system associated with ulcers.

Broccoli Smoothie

Ingredient:

1 cup broccoli florets

1 ripe banana

1/2 cup plain Greek yogurt

3/4 cup almond milk

2 tablespoons honey (optional)

Instructions:

1. Wash and dry the broccoli florets.

2. Peel and chop the banana, then add to a blender with broccoli, yogurt, almond milk, and honey (if desired). Blend until smooth.

3. Taste-test the smoothie and add more honey if desired; blend again.

4. Pour into glasses and enjoy!

This delicious broccoli smoothie is a great source of minerals that can help protect your body from ulcers as well as reduce inflammation associated with existing ulcers. Enjoy it as part of a regular Ulcer Prevention Plan!

Kale Smoothie

Ingredient:

2 cups kale

1 ripe banana

1/2 cup plain Greek yogurt

3/4 cup almond milk

2 tablespoons honey (optional)

Instructions:

1. Wash and dry the kale leaves.

2. Peel and chop the banana, then add to a blender with the kale, yogurt, almond milk, and honey (if desired). Blend until smooth.

3. Taste-test the smoothie and add more honey if desired; blend again.

4. Pour into glasses and enjoy!

Celery Smoothie

Ingredient:

2 celery stalks

1 ripe banana

1/2 cup plain Greek yogurt

3/4 cup almond milk

2 tablespoons honey (optional)

Instructions:

1. Wash and dry the celery stalks.

2. Peel and chop the banana, then add to a blender with celery, yogurt, almond milk, and honey (if desired). Blend until smooth.

3. Taste-test the smoothie and add more honey if desired; blend again.

4. Pour into glasses and enjoy!

Easy Cucumber Smoothie

ingredient :

1 cucumber

1 ripe banana

1/2 cup plain Greek yogurt

3/4 cup almond milk

2 tablespoons honey (optional)

Instructions:

1. Peel and chop the cucumber, then add to a blender along with the banana, yogurt, almond milk, and honey (if desired). Blend until smooth.

2. Taste-test the smoothie and add more honey if desired; blend again.

3. Pour into glasses and enjoy!

This refreshing cucumber smoothie is full of vitamins that can help reduce inflammation associated with ulcers as well as protect against further issues down the line.

Green Veggie Smoothie

ingredient :

1/2 cup kale

1/2 cup spinach

1 ripe banana

1/2 cup plain Greek yogurt

3/4 cup almond milk

2 tablespoons honey (optional)

Instructions:

1. Wash and dry the kale and spinach leaves.

2. Pecl and chop the banana, then add to a blender along with the greens, yogurt, almond milk, and honey (if desired). Blend until smooth.

3. Taste-test the smoothie and add more honey if desired; blend again.

4. Pour into glasses and enjoy!

This delicious green veggie smoothie is packed full of vitamins that can help reduce inflammation associated with ulcers as well as protect against future issues. So enjoy it regularly to help manage and prevent ulcers!

Pumpkin Smoothie

ingredient :

1/2 cup canned pumpkin

1 ripe banana

1/2 cup plain Greek yogurt

3/4 cup almond milk

2 tablespoons honey (optional)

Instructions:

1. Add the canned pumpkin to a blender along with the banana, yogurt, almond milk, and honey (if desired). Blend until smooth.

2. Taste-test the smoothie and add more honey if desired; blend again.

3. Pour into glasses and enjoy!

This tasty pumpkin smoothie is filled with vitamins and minerals that can help reduce inflammation in your digestive system associated with ulcers as well as provide protection against future issues. Enjoy

Avocado Smoothie

ingredient :

1/2 avocado

1 ripe banana

1/2 cup plain Greek yogurt

3/4 cup almond milk

2 tablespoons honey (optional)

Instructions:

1. Peel and chop the avocado, then add to a blender along with the banana, yogurt, almond milk, and honey (if desired). Blend until smooth.

2. Taste-test the smoothie and add more honey if desired; blend again.

3. Pour into glasses and enjoy!

This creamy avocado smoothie is full of vitamins that can help reduce inflammation associated with ulcers as well as provide protection against further issues down the line.

DAIRY SMOOTHIES

Coconut Milk Smoothie

ingredient :

-1 cup coconut milk

-1 banana (preferably frozen)

-2 tablespoons of honey

-1/4 teaspoon ground ginger

This simple smoothie is a delicious way to get the healing benefits of coconut milk. Coconut milk has anti-inflammatory properties and can help reduce ulcer pain, soothe the digestive system, and protect against further damage. The banana and honey provide sweetness that helps make this drink enjoyable while also delivering extra nutrients such as vitamin B6, potassium, magnesium, manganese, and iron.

Finally, ground ginger adds an extra layer of protection by stimulating saliva production which can help reduce inflammation and speed up healing.

Oat Milk Smoothie

ingredient :

-1 cup oat milk

-1/2 cup frozen spinach or kale

-1 banana (preferably frozen)

-1/4 teaspoon ground cinnamon

-Pinch of nutmeg

Oats are a great source of soluble fiber, which can help reduce ulcer pain and protect the digestive system. If you're looking for a dairy alternative, oat milk makes an excellent choice in smoothie recipes. The addition of nutrient-rich green vegetables adds even more healing benefits while the spices provide flavor and add anti-inflammatory properties. Cinnamon helps to soothe inflammation while nutmeg aids digestion and relieves pain associated with stomach ulcers

Almond Milk Smoothie

ingredient :

-1 cup almond milk

-1/2 cup frozen blueberries or blackberries

-1 banana (preferably frozen)

-2 tablespoons of honey

Almond milk is an excellent source of healthy fats, proteins, and antioxidants that can help reduce ulcer symptoms and protect against further damage. The addition of fresh or frozen berries provides a boost of fiber as well as important vitamins and minerals while the honey helps to sweeten the smoothie. This delicious recipe is a great way to get all the healing benefits of almond milk in one delicious drink!

Dairy-Free Spinach Smoothie

ingredient :

-1 cup coconut milk

-2 cups spinach, fresh or frozen

-1 banana (preferably frozen)

-2 tablespoons of honey

-Pinch of ground turmeric

Spinach is an excellent source of vitamin A and many other important nutrients that can help heal existing ulcers and protect against future issues. This dairy-free smoothie combines the healing benefits of spinach with the anti-inflammatory properties of turmeric and coconut milk. The sweet flavor of the banana and honey makes this drink enjoyable while also providing additional vitamins and minerals for maximum health benefits. Enjoy this delicious recipe as a tasty way to get all the healing benefits you need!

Acai Smoothie

ingredient :

-1 acai smoothie pack or 2 tablespoons of dried acai powder

-1 cup almond milk

-1 banana (preferably frozen)

-2 tablespoons of honey

-Pinch of ground cinnamon

Acai is a superfood that is packed with vitamins, minerals, and antioxidants that can help reduce ulcer pain and support the body's natural healing process. This smoothie combines the power of acai with almond milk for an ultra-nutritious drink. The banana and honey provide sweetness while the cinnamon adds an extra layer of protection against inflammation and helps to soothe digestive issues.

Glowing Green Smoothie

ingredient :

-1 cup coconut milk

-2 cups spinach, fresh or frozen

-1/2 cup kale leaves

-1 banana (preferably frozen)

-2 tablespoons of honey

-Pinch of ground ginger

This glowing green smoothie is packed with vitamins and minerals that can help reduce ulcer symptoms and promote healing. The combination of spinach, kale, and coconut milk provides a powerful blend of anti-inflammatory properties while the banana and honey add sweetness to make it enjoyable. Finally, ground ginger adds an extra layer of protection by stimulating saliva production which can help reduce inflammation and speed up healing. Enjoy this delicious recipe for a healthy way to heal your body!

Dairy Free Peanut Butter Smoothie

ingredient :

-1 cup almond milk

-2 tablespoons of natural peanut butter

-1 banana (preferably frozen)

-2 tablespoons of honey

-Pinch of ground cinnamon

This dairy-free smoothie is packed with healthy fats and proteins that can help soothe existing ulcers and provide protection against future issues. The combination of almond milk, peanut butter, and banana provides an excellent source of fiber as well as important vitamins and minerals for a healthy digestive system.

Dairy Free Mango Smoothie

ingredient :

-1 cup coconut milk

-2 cups frozen mango

-2 tablespoons of honey

-Pinch of ground ginger

This dairy-free smoothie is an excellent source of vitamins, minerals, and antioxidants that can help reduce ulcer symptoms and provide protection against further damage. The combination of coconut milk and frozen mango provides a delicious flavor while the honey adds sweetness to make it even more enjoyable. Finally, the addition of ground ginger helps to stimulate saliva production, which can help reduce inflammation and speed up healing. Enjoy this delicious smoothie for a healthy way to heal your body!

Avocado Banana Smoothie

ingredient :

-1 cup coconut milk

-1/2 avocado

-1 banana (preferably frozen)

-2 tablespoons of honey

-Pinch of ground cinnamon

This creamy avocado banana smoothie is an excellent source of vitamins, minerals, and healthy fats that can help soothe existing ulcers and provide protection against future issues. The combination of coconut milk and avocado makes this drink ultra-nourishing while the banana adds sweetness to make it even more enjoyable.

Dairy-Free Kale Smoothie

ingredient :

-1 cup almond milk

-2 cups kale leaves

-1 banana (preferably frozen)

-2 tablespoons of honey

-Pinch of ground ginger

This dairy-free kale smoothie is an excellent source of vitamins, minerals, and antioxidants that can help reduce inflammation and promote healing. The combination of almond milk, kale, and banana provides a powerful blend of anti-inflammatory properties while the honey adds sweetness to make it enjoyable.

Beet Smoothie

ingredient :

-1 cup coconut milk

-1/2 cup cooked beets

-1 banana (preferably frozen)

-2 tablespoons of honey

-Pinch of ground cinnamon.

This beet smoothie is packed with vitamins, minerals, and antioxidants that can help reduce ulcer symptoms and promote healing. The combination of coconut milk, beets, and banana provides a delicious flavor while the honey adds sweetness to make it even more enjoyable.

Celery Smoothie

ingredient :

-1 cup almond milk

-2 stalks celery

-1 banana (preferably frozen)

-2 tablespoons of honey

-Pinch of ground ginger

This celery smoothie is packed with vitamins and minerals that can help reduce ulcer symptoms and promote healing. The combination of almond milk, celery, and banana provides an excellent source of fiber as well as important nutrients for a healthy digestive system.

Dairy-Free Fruit Smoothie

ingredient :

-1 cup coconut milk

-2 cups frozen mixed berries

-1 banana (preferably frozen)

-2 tablespoons of honey

-Pinch of ground cinnamon

This dairy-free fruit smoothie is packed with vitamins, minerals, and antioxidants that can help reduce ulcer symptoms and provide protection against further damage.

HIGH- FIBER SMOOTHIES

Avocado Pineapple High-Fiber Smoothie

ingredient :

- 1/2 cup of chopped pineapple

- 1/2 ripe avocado

- 1 teaspoon of honey

- 2 tablespoons of chia seeds

- 3/4 cup coconut milk

instructions:

1. Place all the ingredients in a blender and blend until smooth.

2. Pour the mixture into a glass and enjoy!

Peaches & Cream Oatmeal Smoothie

ingredient :

- 1/2 cup of frozen peaches

- 1/4 cup of rolled oats

- 2 tablespoons of honey

- 1 teaspoon of vanilla extract

- 3/4 cup coconut milk

instructions:

1. Place the peaches, oats, honey, vanilla extract, and coconut milk into a blender and blend until smooth.

2. Pour the mixture into a glass and enjoy!

best High-Fiber Smoothie for Constipation and Bloating

ingredient :

- 1/2 cup of raspberries

- 1/4 cup of plain yogurt

- 2 tablespoons of honey

- 2 tablespoons of chia seeds

- 3/4 cup coconut milk

instructions:

1. Place all the ingredients in a blender and blend until smooth.

2. Pour the mixture into a glass and enjoy!

These smoothies are packed with vitamins, minerals, and other important nutrients that can help soothe existing ulcers and prevent future issues. Drinking these smoothies on a regular basis can also help with constipation and bloating, as well as provide your body with essential fiber to keep your gut healthy. Enjoy!

High-Fiber Detox Smoothie

ingredient :

- 1/2 cup of blueberries

- 1/4 cup of plain yogurt

- 2 tablespoons of honey

- 1 teaspoon of turmeric powder

- 3/4 cup coconut milk

instructions:

1. Place all the ingredients in a blender and blend until smooth.

2. Pour the mixture into a glass and enjoy!

This High-Fiber Detox Smoothie is packed with antioxidants from the blueberries, probiotics from the yogurt, and anti-inflammatory properties from the turmeric. Not only will this help with ulcers but also promote gut health and detoxify your body of any toxic buildup. Enjoy!

High-Fiber Smoothie for Gut Health

ingredient :

- 1/2 cup of strawberries

- 1/4 cup of plain yogurt

- 2 tablespoons of honey

- 2 tablespoons of psyllium husk powder

- 3/4 cup coconut milk

instructions:

1. Place all the ingredients in a blender and blend until smooth.

2. Pour the mixture into a glass and enjoy!

This High-Fiber Smoothie for Gut Health is packed with probiotics from the yogurt, vitamins from the strawberries, and fiber from the psyllium husk powder to promote digestion, reduce inflammation, and make sure your gut stays healthy. Enjoy!

Jackfruit Smoothie

ingredient :

- 1/2 cup of jackfruit

- 1/4 cup of plain yogurt

- 2 tablespoons of honey

- 1 teaspoon of flaxseed oil

- 3/4 cup coconut milk

instructions:

1. Place all the ingredients in a blender and blend until smooth.

2. Pour the mixture into a glass and enjoy!

This Jackfruit Smoothie is packed with fiber, probiotics, vitamins, minerals and omega fatty acids that are important for promoting good gut health and reducing inflammation. Enjoy!

High-Fiber Vegan Smoothie

ingredient :

- 1/2 cup of mango

- 1/4 cup of almond milk

- 2 tablespoons of honey

- 2 tablespoons of hemp seeds

- 3/4 cup coconut milk

instructions:

1. Place all the ingredients in a blender and blend until smooth.

2. Pour the mixture into a glass and enjoy!

This High-Fiber Vegan Smoothie is packed with vitamins, minerals and other essential nutrients from the mango, protein from the hemp seeds, and probiotics from the almond milk to promote good gut health while providing natural relief for existing ulcers. Enjoy!

Pear Smoothie

ingredient :

- 1/2 cup of pears

- 1/4 cup of plain yogurt

- 2 tablespoons of honey

- 2 tablespoons of chia seeds

- 3/4 cup coconut milk

instructions:

1. Place all the ingredients in a blender and blend until smooth.

2. Pour the mixture into a glass and enjoy!

This Pear Smoothie is packed with vitamins from the pears, probiotics from the yogurt, omega fatty acids from the chia seeds, and fiber to help promote good gut health. Enjoy!

High-Fiber Smoothie with Beetroot

ingredient :

- 1/2 cup of beetroot

- 1/4 cup of almond milk

- 2 tablespoons of honey

- 1 teaspoon of ginger powder

- 3/4 cup coconut milk

instructions:

1. Place all the ingredients in a blender and blend until smooth.

2. Pour the mixture into a glass and enjoy!

This High-Fiber Smoothie with Beetroot is packed with vitamins, minerals, and other essential nutrients from the beetroot, protein from the almond milk, and anti-inflammatory properties from the ginger to help soothe existing ulcers while also boosting your overall gut health. Enjoy!

Easy Flax Seed Smoothie

ingredient :

- 1/2 cup of pineapple

- 1/4 cup of plain yogurt

- 2 tablespoons of honey

- 1 tablespoon of ground flax seed

- 3/4 cup coconut milk

instructions:

1. Place all the ingredients in a blender and blend until smooth.

2. Pour the mixture into a glass and enjoy!

This Easy Flax Seed Smoothie is packed with antioxidants from the pineapple, probiotics from the yogurt, omega fatty acids from the flax seed to promote good gut health as well as provide natural relief for existing ulcers. Enjoy!

Apple Cinnamon Smoothie

ingredient :

- 1/2 cup of apples

- 1/4 cup of almond milk

- 2 tablespoons of honey

- 1 teaspoon of cinnamon powder

- 3/4 cup coconut milk

instructions:

1. Place all the ingredients in a blender and blend until smooth.

2. Pour the mixture into a glass and enjoy!

This Apple Cinnamon Smoothie is packed with vitamins, minerals, and other essential nutrients from the apple, protein from the almond milk, and anti-inflammatory properties from the cinnamon to help soothe existing ulcers while boosting your overall gut health. Enjoy!

HERBAL SMOOTHIES

Ashwagandha Banana and Almond Butter Smoothie

Ingredients

- 1 banana, frozen
- 1 cup oat milk, unsweetened
- 1/4 cup raw almond butter

- 1 tablespoon Ashwagandha powder
- 1 teaspoon cinnamon powder
- A dash of honey (only if you'd like to add a hint of sweetness)

Directions

Place ingredients in a blender and blend until smooth! Serve immediately

Calming Cherry Chamomile Smoothie

Ingredients

- 1 cup coconut milk
- 1/2 cup cold chamomile tea
- 1 cup frozen cherries
- 1 cup frozen mangos
- 1 teaspoon flax seeds
- 1 tablespoon coconut oil
- A few drops of liquid stevia
- 1 teaspoon of pure vanilla extract (optional)

Directions

Place ingredients in a blender and blend until smooth! Serve immediately.

Lavender and Wild Blueberry Smoothie

Ingredients

- 1 cup of frozen wild blueberries
- 1/2 banana
- 1/2 avocado
- 1/2 cup cold lavender tea
- 1 cup of your favorite plant-based milk of choice
- 1 teaspoon of pure vanilla extract
- A few drops of liquid stevia (optional)
- 1/2 cup of ice

Directions

Place ingredients in a blender and blend until smooth! Serve immediately.

CONCLUSION

Smoothies can be an important part of any ulcer management plan. Not only do they provide essential nutrients, but they also help to reduce stress and improve digestion. Drinking smoothies regularly can help prevent future ulcers and support the healing process of existing ones. Make sure to use organic ingredients when possible and include a variety of fruits, vegetables, and proteins in your smoothie recipes for maximum benefit. With regular consumption of smoothies, you can enjoy improved health while protecting yourself against ulcers.